Essential Oils

Transform your Life with Essential Oils & Aromatherapy. DIY Almond Oil Recipes for Natural Beauty, Gifts and Curing Illnesses

Jonathan S. Hunt

Contents

Chapter 1. What It Is & An Almond Oil Overview

Almond oil is a great oil for your hair, skin and health. There are many beneficial properties as well as nutrients, and it's considered to be a great ingredient for homemade cosmetics as well. It compares to many skin care products, and almond oil doesn't have any side effects that you have to worry about. One of the main uses of almond oil is to give your skin that healthy glow you want while making sure that you get rid of anything that's marring it, including dark circles. Sweet almond oil is able to ingested, and you can put it in a variety of herbal remedies to make sure that you are using it for all of its benefits.

So What Is It?

It's an oil that's literally extracted from almonds, and remember that there are actually different types of almonds, but they usually are in two classes. There are your bitter almonds, and they're bitter when you eat them, so very few people will actually use them in a recipe or eat them on their own. However, you can get bitter almond oil from them, and you'll find it has a little hydrogen cyanide in it, which is poisonous, so you can't eat it. Eating bitter almonds can lead to vertigo, even if you've only eaten a few. It can even kill you, so they're not meant to be ingested.

Then there are sweet almonds, and these are the ones that people eat, and they taste great. They have a sweet taste, and the oil that is made from them is sweet in it taste as well. Almonds actually aren't nuts, but they're called a drupe. The US produces most of the almonds, and most of them come from California. There are subtle differences in the varieties of sweet almonds, but it doesn't matter that much for its benefits.

Some Properties:

You may be wondering what properties that almond oil really has, and the fact is that almond oil is a great way to deal with many problems. For example anti-inflammatory, which means that it can reduce any inflammation that you're experiencing if you take it orally or topically. It even has many antioxidants, and it'll help to boost your immune system. It can even boot your immune system if it's done topically. Of course an internal application is known to work better if you're using it as an immune booster to help protect against various diseases.

Almond oil is also known as an anti-hepatotoxic, which will help you eliminate toxins in your liver, and it's very similar to castor oil in this way. It's also a laxative, so you won't have to worry about constipation if you're taking it regularly. Of course, it's only a mild laxative, and it's an emollient when applied topically. You won't have to deal with dry skin anymore if you're using it topically.

As a sclerosant, you'll find that it can help with spider veins, varicose veins and even hemorrhoids, and it's an analgesic, which makes it a pain reliever. Just keep in mind that it's only a mild pain reliever. It'll help with a variety of conditions, and there are many different ways to use it.

Some Common Benefits:

You may be wondering what some common benefits are, and using it for your skin is one of them. It'll even help your skin to be a little less dull. It can help with chapped lips as well. Eczema and psoriasis are also a thing of the past if you're using almond oil on a regular basis. Of course, it's commonly a massage oil as well. Even massage therapists will commonly use almond oil because of its benefits to your skin. It even spreads easily, and it's an oil that will absorb into your oil but not too quickly, allowing you to really work it into your pores and over the area. This way you don't have to reapply it too often while receiving or giving a massage with almond oil.

Almond oil can commonly be used for your hair and face as well. It reduce sagging and even wrinkles, helping to make sure that you don't feel the effects of aging as badly. You can just apply it directly to your skin on a regular basis to brighten up your skin and help to soothe out any fine lines that's bothering you. Almond oil has been used since ancient times, and it has been mentioned in many herbalist texts. Because of its versatility, it's commonly used in various recipes, remedies, and treatments that are going to make you feel and look better.

Chapter 2. Using It for Cosmetics & Beauty

Almond oils is great for cosmetics. One of the main reasons is that it's great at reducing inflammation that can damage your skin, and it can even help to heal your skin. This leads to anti-aging properties that are sure to help you look even better. It can treat numerous hair and beauty issues. It's high in vitamin E as well as having many antioxidants that will benefit your skin and hair.

Use #1 Remove Too Much Tan:

You don't have to worry about getting too dark if you're being careful and have almond oil around. Almond oil is going to help lighten your skin, and that means that if you get too tan, you're going to want to have almond oil on hand. Lighten yourself by a few shades by applying almond oil directly to your tanned skin, and it'll help you to look like you want to. However, this remedy will help a little more than just almond oil alone. The lime juice is known to help lighten it, and the milk and honey is also going to help to moisturize your skin to keep it from drying out. Drying it out is a common problem if you've tanned too much.

Ingredients:

1. 1 Tablespoon Honey, Raw

2. 3 Tablespoons Almond Oil

3. 1 Teaspoon Lime Juice

4. 3-4 Teaspoons Milk Powder

Direction:

1. Mix everything into a clean bowl, and then apply it to the areas that you think is too dark. This is commonly your face.

2. Let it sit for fifteen to twenty minutes before washing it with cool water.

3. Pat it dry gently, and then reapply once daily until you're at the tone you want.

Use #2 A Makeup Remover

A lot of makeup removers are actually too harsh for your skin, and that's why it's important that you use something that will make sure it doesn't damage your skin. The solution is almond oil. It's a light option that won't leave grease behind, and better yet, it's great on sensitive skin as well, which most makeup removers just aren't. It works best because it'll open up your pores to make sure that no makeup is left behind in them, which could later cause blackheads and acne if not removed. It works for almost all skin types as well.

Ingredients:

1. 1 Teaspoon Almond Oil

2. A Cotton Ball

Directions:

1. Take the almond oil and place it in a clean bowl, and then dip in the cotton ball.

2. Gently remove the makeup with the slightly damp cotton ball.

3. Then, it's best to wash and dry your face with cool water.

Use #3 Simple & Shiny Hair

Shiny hair can be simple. Of course, there are complex remedies for shiny hair as well, which are known to work a little better because it works on different levels. Of course, sometimes this simple one ingredient recipe does the trick. You just need to know when to apply it.

Ingredients:

1.   2 Teaspoons Almond Oil

Directions:

1. You'll need more or less depending on if your hair is thick, thin, short or long.

2. Make sure not to apply too much almond oil to your hair, and only apply it after its wet, as that's the best time.

3. Then, let it dry by only applying it to the shaft of your hair and then wait. Do this after you shower every day, and you'll have shinier hair.

Use #4 Detangle Your Hair

If your hair is too dry, then it's more likely to tangle up, and this can cause it to be frizzy when it dries. It'll be hard to brush through, and you're more likely to get split ends that will make your hair look a mess, and it won't matter if your shampoo was good or not, and sometimes it doesn't even matter out your conditioner. Once again, almond oil can be used to help you with this beauty hack.

Ingredients:

1. 1 Teaspoon Almond Oil

Directions:

1. Apply the almond oil to your comb or hairbrush, and run it through your hair. Do not use the full teaspoon unless you need it, as you don't want to drench your hair in almond oil. You should be able to brush through your hair much easily as it helps to detangle for you.

Use #5 Treating Dark Circles

You don't need to deal with dark circles anymore, and this almond oil treatment is sure to help you get rid of them quickly. Getting rid of them quickly is important, but try to skip the cover up as it can be counterproductive. It's hard when you're still dealing with the circles, but you'll get rid of them faster overall if you're making sure that you use natural remedies without chemicals getting in the way.

Ingredients:

1. 3 Teaspoons Almond Oil

2. 3 Teaspoons Aloe Vera Gel

Directions:

1. Take a small clean bottle and combine the aloe vera gel and the almond oil. Make sure it's completely mixed.

2. You'll have to shake it before every use, but you can put it up for future use.

3. Put a small bit in a cotton ball and use it like you would makeup remover on your dark circles. Do this two to three times daily. You will notice results within two to three days, but you may need to keep applying for a week or more.

Use #6 Homemade Moisturizer

If you're looking for a way to moisturize your skin on a deeper level than just applying the almond oil directly, then this cream is for you. It's even easy to use. Rosewater even acts a toner, and it's easy to make if you don't want to buy it as well. This is a moisturizer that you make up in advance, so make sure that you have an airtight container that you can store it in so that it stays good. You'll even be able to take it with you to apply throughout the day.

Ingredients:

1. 4 Ounces Rosewater

2. 8 Tablespoons Beeswax, Grated

3. 200 ml Sweet Almond Oil

4. 1 Tablespoon Honey, Raw

Directions:

1. Melt your almond oil and beeswax together over low heat in a double boiler.

2. Add in your honey, making sure it's mixed.

3. Add in your rosewater, and mix well. Then, let it cool, putting it into airtight containers for later use. Store out of sunlight in a cool, dry place.

Use #7 Almond Oil Facemask

The almond oil is going to help with any and all dry skin problems as well as wrinkles, but the banana is going to help as well. It has vitamin B,

E and even A in it that is great for your skin, and they're anti-aging. It's also known to help exfoliate skin which will remove the dead skin that has your face looking dull. The egg has vitamin B2, B3 and even zinc which is good for your skin as well. It'll help with stress and acne. It'll also help to tighten your skin and give you a facelift.

Ingredients:

1. 1 Egg Yolk

2. 2 Teaspoons Sweet Almond Oil

3. 1 Small Banana, Ripe

Directions:

1. Make sure that your banana is peeled and mashed.

2. Bea the egg yolk to make it fluffy, and then beat the almond oil in as well.

3. Mix in the banana, and apply to your face.

4. Leave for ten to fifteen minutes, and then wash it off with cool water, patting it dry.

Use #8 Strengthen Your Nails

Everyone wants strong nails, and you can't always get strong nails by just hoping for them. This is why you should try to make sure that you are actively trying to make your nails shine. Just take a little almond oil, and applying it right and regularly will do the trick.

Ingredients:

1. ½ Teaspoon Almond Oil

Directions:

1. Make sure that your nails are trimmed and filed, and then you can rub the almond oil into the skin around them as well as the nails themselves.

2. Do this two to three times daily, and you'll notice stronger, shinier nails within a few days, but longer lasting results will come with time.

Use #9 Lengthen Lashes

You can lengthen your lashes with almond oil as well. You don't have to try and buy mascara to hide thin eyelashes, and you can get the lashes you always wanted naturally. Just take an empty mascara bottle and clean it out, as it'll help you to get something to apply it in, but other bottles will work as well if you're careful. The castor oil is full of omega 6 fatty acids, and it even has proteins and vitamin E oil. The sweet almond oil will moisturize it, and the vitamin E oil will strengthen it. Together, you'll have full lashes in no time at all.

Ingredients:

1. 3 Parts Castor Oil

2. 1/8 Part Sweet Almond Oil

3. 1/8 Part Vitamin E Oil

Directions:

1. Just mix it all together and shake. Apply to your lashes at least once daily.

Use #10 Hot Oil Treatments

Hot oil treatments are great for your hair, and it'll give you the full body shine that you could want. So it's important that you find a cheap alternative to any chemical laden hot oil treatments out there. All you need is almond oil.

Ingredients:

1. ¼ Cup Sweet Almond Oil

Directions:

1. Take and heat up the almond oil like you would for any hot oil treatment, and then apply it to your scalp.

2. Cover with a shower cap, and let it sit for two three hours.

3. Wash out.

Chapter 3. Miracle Uses for Skin Conditions

There are many skin conditions that can be helped with almond oil. Sweet almond oil is great to use, and it's extremely versatile. It's easy to use, and even easier to get ahold of. You don't have to deal with eczema, psoriasis, ringworms or other skin conditions anymore, and you can skip the over the counter medication and prescription drugs.

Cure #1 Ringworm Help

Almond oil is going to help you with ringworm, but it's not enough on its own. You need the right essential oil to help out, but almond oil is antibacterial on its own, which is going to help speed the process along. It'll also help with cell regeneration, which is needed if you're healing from any skin condition. Skip the over the counter cream and the tea tree oil will help because it's an antifungal. Many people are too sensitive to tea tree oil when it's applied directly to your skin, and that's why the almond oil acts as a carrier oil, making it safe. The lemongrass essential oil is used for the same reason as the tea tree oil.

Ingredients:

1. ½ Teaspoon Almond Oil

2. 4-5 Drops Tea Tree Oil

3. 5-8 Drops Lemongrass Oil

Directions:

1. Wash and dry the area with cool water.

2. Mix all ingredients together in a clean bowl.

3. Gently take a cotton ball and dip it into the mixture, applying liberally to the area.

4. Cover with gauze and reapply three times daily.

Cure #2 Toenail Fungus

Almond oil is great for your skin and nails, and it'll keep the strong and healthy. It can rescue them as well. Its immune boosting abilities as its anti-inflammatory abilities comes in handy with this wonderful remedy. Add in the tea tree oil for its antifungal properties, and sweet almond oil can help you with your toenail fungus problem as well.

Ingredients:

1. 1 Teaspoon Sweet Almond Oil

2. 5-8 Drops Tea Tree Oil

Directions:

1. Wash the area, and then take a clean bowl to mix your ingredients.

2. Apply liberally to the area with a cotton ball, and let it dry on the affected area.

3. Reapply three to four times daily.

Cure #3 General Rashes

You may not always know what your rash is from, but almond oil can help you to get rid of most rashes. If a rash persists, remember to contact your doctor. Almond oil will reduce any inflammation that comes with your rash, but it will also help with soothing the skin and helping cell regeneration. Its boost to your immune system will help your body fight off the rash naturally. The peppermint oil will sooth the rash as well as it has antifungal and antibacterial qualities.

Ingredients:

1. 1 Tablespoon Almond Oil

2. 4-6 Drops Peppermint Oil

Directions:

1. Mix everything together in a clean bowl, and then apply to the area.

2. Let it dry on, and do it two to three times per day.

3. If improvement is not seen in three to four days, contact your doctor.

Cure #4 Stretch Mark Reducer

Almond oil will help your skin shine and regenerate at a cellular level. That's why it's so important to use it if you feel uncomfortable with any stretch marks. It's easier if you're doing it at the start of stretch marks, but even when it's already there, you can get rid of your stretch marks easily. Lemon juice brightens the skin, and with the almond oil you don't have to worry about your skin drying out. This will also help to reduce stretch marks.

Ingredients:

1. 1 Teaspoon Almond Oil

2. ½ Teaspoon Fresh Lemon Juice

Directions:

1. Mix everything together in a fresh bowl, and then apply it to the area. You can do this using your fingers or a cotton ball.

2. Let it sit and soak in. rub it in using circular motions, making sure to get the entire area.

Cure #5 Eczema Help

If you live with eczema, you already know that it can be both embarrassing as well as painful if you let it get to bad. Sometimes, over the counter creams and prescription drugs don't work, and a natural solution will help you to skip all of the side effects. Eczema can be helped through almond oil, and partly because of the vitamin E, but also because of the anti-inflammatory effects that almond oil has. When you pair it with lavender essential oil, you have an eczema cure that is sure to help. It's antibacterial and antiseptic, helping to get rid of your eczema in a heartbeat.

Ingredients:

1. 1 Tablespoon Almond Oil

2. 8-12 Drops Lavender Oil

Directions:

1. Mix everything together.

2. After washing and drying the area gently, apply the mixture and let it soak in. many people will cover it with a gauze pad to give it time to work.

3. Reapply two to three times daily. After one to two days you should see improvement.

Cure #6 Helping with Psoriasis

Almond oil can help with psoriasis for the same reasons that it can help with eczema. The two are very similar, but you'll need a different essential oil. Thyme oil can be helpful because it's an antiseptic, which helps it with psoriasis, but it cannot be used without a carrier oil or you will feel a sting. Geranium oil is added in because it helps to revitalize the tissue.

Ingredients:

1. 1 Teaspoon Almond Oil

2. 6-8 Drops Geranium Oil

3. 8-10 Drops Thyme Oil

Directions:

1. Mix everything together, and make sure to use cool water to wash and dry the area.

2. Apply the mixture, and cover with gauze. Reapply three to four times daily.

Cure #7 Acne Scars

Acne is hard enough, but when you have acne scars you're going to want to lessen them or get rid of them completely. This is where almond oil can once again be your miracle cure. Lemon juice, when fresh, is going to help to brighten the skin and help to erase the way that acne scars stand out. The almond oil is going to make sure that it stays moisturized and your skin heals on its own. The aloe vera gel is going to help to lighten the scar as well and provides many antioxidants.

Ingredients:

1. 1 Teaspoon Sweet Almond Oil

2. ½ Teaspoon Aloe Vera Gel

3. ½ Teaspoon Lemon Juice, Fresh

Directions:

1. Mix all of the ingredients together thoroughly in a clean bowl.

2. Apply liberally to the area and let it soak in and dry. Do this at least once or twice daily for the best results.

Repetition:

Remember that repetition is really what makes the difference when you're using any of these treatments involving almond oil for skin conditions. This is because nothing is going to be healed with one application. You shouldn't expect to see results until after three applications. It may take as long as 4 days before results are seen. Remember to get any and all rashes checked out by your doctor, and if you have a negative reaction o almond oil, contact your doctor immediately.

Chapter 4. Useful Almond Oil Cream Recipes

There are many different creams that you can make from almond oil for various ailments and uses. Of course, these creams take a little more time than the almond oil uses that have been previously listed, but they store for quite some time and area usually made up in advance. Just remember to store them in a cool, dark place, and all creams should be in an airtight container. It's best to store them in glass containers, as it'll help to make sure that none of the ingredients interact with plastic, which could change the composition of the cream you're using and therefore its results. Small mason jars are recommended, but tin containers are usually okay as well.

Cream #1 Simple Facial Moisturizer

It's important to keep your face looking young and healthy, and that's what a facial moisturizer is for. This one is easy to make, and almond oil is one of its main ingredients. It can store for a few months. The aloe vera gel is actually going to help because of how antioxidant rich it is, and the beeswax is mainly used for its consistency help. Lavender essential oil is relaxing, and so it should help to keep stress lines away as well as it can help to lighten and improve your skin. Coconut oil also has vitamin E.

Ingredients:

1. ¼ Cup Sweet Almond Oil

2. ¼ Cup Coconut Oil

3. 1 Cup Aloe Vera Gel

4. 10-15 Drops Lavender Essential Oil

5. ¾ Ounce Beeswax, Grated

Directions:

1. Take a double boiler and met together your beeswax and oils.

2. Mix in your aloe vera gel, and then remove from heat.

3. While cooling, mix in your lavender essential oil and store in airtight containers.

Cream #2 Anti-Wrinkle Cream

If you're worried about the effects of aging, you shouldn't have to worry any longer. Not if you have almond oil in your home. It's best to buy it in bulk, especially if you're making various creams from it. Almond oil is rejuvenating and will keep you young, but it's only one of the helpful ingredients in this cream recipe. The rosehip seed oil is also important because of its vitamin A, which will help to reduce the depth of wrinkles. It'll even boost the speed at which your cells regrow, which will help you stay looking youthful. Coconut oil is great to moisturize and revitalize your skin, and lemon oil will help to both lighten dark spots and reduce wrinkles.

Ingredients:

1. ½ Ounce Beeswax

2. 2 Tablespoons Coconut Oil

3. 2 Tablespoons Sweet Almond Oil

4. ½ Teaspoon Lemon Essential Oil

5. ½ Teaspoon Rosehip Seed Oil

Directions:

1. Take a double boiler, melting your sweet almond oil and coconut oil with your beeswax.

2. Take off heat and put it into a bowl. As it cools, mix in your essential oils.

3. Put into a separate container for later use. It's best to use at least once or twice daily for the best results.

Cream #3 Shaving Cream

You don't have to deal with dry or itchy skin after shaving any longer. This is a great cream no matter if you're a man or a woman, and it keeps for quite some time. The almond oil will make sure that your skin stays smooth and moist, and with it whipped, it's easy to spread. The shea butter makes it smooth and easy to apply, and the coconut oil will help to keep you looking young.

Ingredients:

1. 1/3 Cup Shea Butter

2. 1/3 Cup Almond Oil

3. ¼ Cup Olive Oil

Directions:

1. Add everything together, meting it in a double boiler. Make sure to stir to make

sure that the shea butter does not get grainy.

2. Remove from heat and put into a bowl. Let cool and turn solid.

3. Whip it until it gets light and fluffy, and then proceed to put it into bowls.

Cream #4 A Salve for Your Hair

Sometimes almond oil isn't enough for your hair, and you're actually going to want to heal split ends with a bit of a salve, which is easy to make if you follow this recipe. You can even use it on your skin and lips. It's perfectly safe, and it'll make your lips soft and lush.

Ingredients:

1. ½ Cup Water, Cooled

2. 1 Tablespoons Glycerin

3. ¼ Cup Sweet Almond Oil

4. ¾ Cup Coconut Oil

5. 2 Tablespoons Olive Oil

Directions:

1. You're going to go want to make or use a double boiler, and melt the coconut oil over it.

2. It should sit and cool for about thirty minutes, and then you can add in the

almond oil, making sure it's whisked together well.

3. Let the mixture sit in the fridge to set for twenty to twenty-five minutes.

4. Make sure to whisk again, and the mixture should be turning into a thick cream.

5. Add a tablespoon of glycerin, and then a half a cup of cooled water.

6. Take the mixture and then continue to whip. You should be able to whip it until it's fluffy, and you can even add a soap color if you want. Do not use another type of dye, though.

7. Spoon into jars to keep. It should have an airtight lid, and tin or glass containers usually work best.

8. You can then either rub it in with your fingers, or you can make a conditioning spray where you make a half and half

mixture of water and the salve, spraying it on your hair.

Cream #5 For Cracked Nipples

This is more of a problem if you're breast feeding but there are rashes that you can get that will crack your nipples if you're a girl as well. Even men can occasionally get cracked nipples, but it's a lot rarer. However, no matter the reason, if you're suffering from cracked nipples this is a salve that will help with the pain and promote healing. Remember that if you're breastfeeding it is important to use only high quality oils, as your baby will come in contact with the residue on your nipples, meaning they should be safe for internal use.

Ingredients:

1. 1 Tablespoon Coconut Oil

2. 2 Tablespoons Sweet Almond Oil

3. 2-4 Drops Lavender Essential Oil

4. 2 Tablespoons Olive Oil

5. 4 Tablespoons Cocoa Butter

Directions:

1. Put your cocoa butter in to heat over a double boiler, adding your olive, coconut, and sweet almond oil as well. Mix together.

2. Take it off heat, and as it begins to cool add in your lavender essential oil.

3. Put into small containers to cool, and use as needed.

Cream #6 Anti-Aging Eye Cream

Anti-aging cream can make your eyes feel and look a little better. There's no reason that you have to worry about dark spots or puffy eyes, and this is an almond oil solution that is easy to make. You can apply it every day, and you'll stay looking young and youthful.

Ingredients:

1. 5-6 Drops Lavender Essential Oil

2. 2 Tablespoons Beeswax

3. ½ Teaspoon Honey, Raw

4. 6 Tablespoons Sweet Almond Oil

5. 2 Tablespoons Rosehip Seed Oil

Directions:

1. Take the beeswax and melt it over a
    double boiler, adding in the sweet

almond oil and rosehip seed oil. Make sure to mix it in.

2. Add in the honey and lavender essential oil, making sure to remove it from heat and mix it thoroughly.

3. Apply once daily around the eyes to avoid puffiness. Do not let it get in your eye.

Cream #7 Varicose Vein Reducer

This is a body butter cream that is going to help to reduce the look of varicose veins, and it can even help to make sure that you're not in as much pain that it can cause. It may sound like a dessert when you read the recipes, but it's great for your skin, and it'll make it silky smooth.

Ingredients:

1. 1 Cup Mango Butter

2. 1 Cup Sweet Almond Oil

3. 5-10 Drops Lavender Essential Oil

4. 10-15 Drops Cedar Wood Essential Oil

5. 5-10 Drops Frankincense Essential Oil

Directions:

1. Melt your mango butter and almond oil together. You can do this over a double boiler, but some people will actually do so in the microwave and it won't hurt.

2. Let it cool slightly before mixing in all of your essential oils, and spoon it into airtight containers to seal.

Cream #8 Cracked Skin Salve

Cracked skin can happen anywhere, and sometimes a nipple cream won't work for rougher skin in the first place. This is great for cracked heels and even cracked hands. It'll make your skin heal as well as just generally smoother and softer.

Ingredients:

1. 1 Ounce Grated Beeswax

2. 1 Ounce Shea Butter

3. 3 Ounces Sweet Almond Oil

4. 2 Ounces Olive Oil

5. ½ Teaspoon Lavender Essential Oil

Directions:

1. Melt the beeswax and the shea butter in a
    double boiler. Remember that you should
    stir constantly if you don't want your shea
    butter to become gritty.

2. Add in the almond oil and olive oil. Stir and remove from heat.

3. Add in the lavender essential oil, making sure that it's mixed in throughout.

4. Place into jars to cool before sealing.

5. To apply just rub it into the area until it sinks in.

Cream #9 All Natural Sunscreen

Just remember that this sunscreen isn't exactly waterproof. You'll need to reapply it every once in a while, but it's much less likely to actually cause any rash. Use a mask for the zinc oxide because it is dangerous to inhale, but fine to be applied to the skin. If you want a thicker sunscreen, then you're going to want to add more beeswax.

Ingredients:

1. ½ Cup Almond Oil

2. ¼ Cup Coconut Oil

3. ¼ Cup Beeswax

4. 2 Tablespoons Zinc Oxide

5. 1 Teaspoon Vitamin E Oil

6. 1 Teaspoon Carrot Seed Oil

7. ½ Teaspoon Vanilla Extract

8. 2 Tablespoons Shea Butter

Directions:

1. You can use an essential oil of your choice rather than vanilla extract if you chose. However, heat up your coconut oil, beeswax, shea butter and almond oil together over a double boiler until smooth and thoroughly mixed.

2. Take off heat, and add in all other oils and extract, mixing thoroughly. Spoon into airtight containers to cool, and then seal.

Chapter 5. Boosting Your Immune System

What most people don't know is that your immune system can be boosted by almond oil as well. Sweet almond can help your immune system, and it can be added simply into your meals. That's one of the best ways to get this benefit. The main reason that almond oil helps with boosting your immune system is its vitamin D. Just remember that you have to use sweet almond oil because bitter almond oil is toxic when ingested.

Vitamin D is needed to stay healthy, and sweet almond oil actually has enough in it to make the difference. Of course, if you don't want to add it into your meals, there are other options. In this chapter you'll find a few drinks and recipes that will help almond oil to help you boost your immune system. Remember that you can also use them by just making sure to replace your cooking oil with almond oil. You can even drizzle it over salads or just take a teaspoon of sweet almond oil every day.

Recipe #1 A Simple Drink

This is a drink that you can drink once daily to help with your immune system, and many people think it tastes pretty good. It's even known to help with other problems, including arthritis because of the turmeric. It's best to drink during the morning time though because this drink is known to bring you a boost of energy as well.

Ingredients:

1. ¼ Cup Water

2. 1/8 Tablespoon Turmeric Powder

3. 1 Cup Goat Milk, Chilled

4. 2 ½ Tablespoon Almond Oil

5. 1 Tablespoon Honey, Raw

Directions:

1. Cook the water and turmeric together for six to eight minutes.

2. Next, make sure to add the milk as well as the almond oil. Bring it to a boil.

3. After it comes to a boil, let it cool down.

4. As it is cooling down, add in your honey, making sure it's fully dissolved. Drink one daily.

Recipe #2 Immune Boosting Smoothie

You can boost your immune system through almond oil by adding it into a smoothie as well. Just make sure it's sweet almond oil, and you can even replace some of the coconut oil in some smoothie recipes to help you make sure you're adding almond oil in. In this smoothie, there are many rich ingredients to help. It can even act as a meal replacement to help aid in a diet change or weight loss.

Ingredients:

1. 2 Tablespoons Almond Butter

2. 1 Tablespoon Almond Oil

3. 1 Medium Banana, Sliced & Frozen

4. 1 Cup Ice

5. ½ Cup Apple Juice, Organic

6. ¼ Cup Blueberries, Frozen

Directions:

1. If you don't have organic apple juice try to make sure that it isn't loaded down with added sugar and sodium.

2. Mix everything together in a blender, and blend until smooth. You can add more almond oil if necessary.

Recipe #3 A Immune Boosting Milk

This is another version of the milk recipe above, and it's going to help make sure your immune system is boosted. If you're using it properly, then you're going to find that the almond oil with the other ingredients included is going to keep you healthy. It can even help to stave off the cold and flu.

Ingredients:

1. 1 Can Coconut Milk, Shaken

2. 1 Teaspoon Cinnamon, Ground

3. ¼ Teaspoon Black Pepper

4. ¼ Teaspoon Cayenne Pepper

5. 1 Teaspoon Turmeric Powder

6. 2 Teaspoons Honey, Raw

7. 2 ½ Tablespoons Sweet Almond Oil

Directions:

1. Take a high speed blender, blending all of the ingredients together until they're smooth.

2. Take a saucepan, putting it over low heat to warm it all up as you pour in the mixture.

3. Drink while still warm.

Recipe #4 Almond Oil Blueberry Pancakes

If you're looking for a breakfast that is going to help you boost your immune system and get through the day, then this is a great almond oil recipe for you. It'll also keep you full and help you start your day on a happier note as well. The blueberries are full of antioxidants, and the almond flour and oil will help along with the raw honey. Local honey is usually best.

Ingredients:

1. ½ Cup Blueberries, Fresh

2. ¼ Cup Goat Milk

3. 2 Tablespoons Honey, Raw

4. 1 ½ Cups Almond Flour, Blanched

5. ¼ Teaspoon Sea Salt, Fine

6. 1 Tablespoon Vanilla Extract

7. ½ Teaspoon Baking Soda

8. 2 Tablespoons Sweet Almond Oil

Directions:

1. Take all of the wet ingredients, whisking them together in a bowl. You'll need a large bowl.

2. All of the dry ingredients should then be added to the wet ingredients, and you'll need to blend.

3. Take a skillet, heating it over low to medium heat, and add in a tablespoon of your almond oil.

4. Take a tablespoon of your batter, and place it in the heated skillet. Sprinkle some blueberries into it.

5. When the pancake begins to bubble, flip it over, and continue to cook until both sides are golden brown.

6. Continue until you are out of batter. Topping with honey will help to boost your immune system a little more as well due to the antioxidants.

Recipe #5 Almond Oil Salad Dressing

If you're eating salad, then you're probably already eating in a healthy manner to keep your immune system out. Of course, adding an almond oil salad dressing is going to help make sure that you're on your way to being a little healthier with a stronger immune system. This one even tastes great.

Feel free to use your own flavor of balsamic vinegar if you don't want raspberry. Add more honey if desired. Raspberries are full of antioxidants, and that will help to make sure that your immune system is boosted as well. The herbs in this recipe are also full of vitamin C which will help.

Ingredients:

1. ¾ Cup Sweet Almond Oil

2. 1 Cup Raspberry Balsamic Vinegar

3. 1 Teaspoon Parsley, Dried

4. 2 Teaspoons Thyme, Dried

5. 1 ½ Teaspoons Rosemary, Dried

6. ½ Teaspoon Honey, Raw

Directions:

1. Take a blender, and blend all ingredients together on high until smooth and completely mixed. Remember that you can use fresh ingredients for your spices as well, but dried is usually easier to get ahold of.

2. Place into a container and keep in the fridge until ready to use. Make sure to shake before each use.

Recipe #6 A Healthy Almond Butter

Almond butter can be used on its own to spread over toast or a bagel, or you can put it in various recipes, including if you're looking for a nut butter for a smoothie. Of course, this is a chocolate almond butter recipe. If you want, you can take out the cocoa powder. Add more or less honey as desired for sweetness. Cocoa powder is also known to help boost your immune system, so long as it is dark cocoa powder. Honey can also help.

Ingredients:

1. 6 ½ lbs Almonds, Raw

2. 3 Tablespoons Sweet Almond Oil

3. 2 Tablespoons Cocoa Powder

4. ½ Teaspoon Honey, Raw

5. ¼ Teaspoon Sea Salt, Fine

Directions:

1. Place everything in the blender, blending on high until it is thoroughly combined.

Recipe #7 Almond Immune Boosting Smoothie

This almond oil smoothie is perfect for breakfast, and it provides vitamin D and vitamin C, which will help to keep you healthy. The ginger is also going to help to boost your immune system, and adding a little bit of rosemary is going to help as well. Fresh rosemary works best, but dried rosemary will work in a pinch. The almond butter helps as well. The blueberries are the main fruit, but with a splash of orange juice and a little coconut oil, you have a nearly tropical blend.

Ingredients:

1. 2 Tablespoons Almond Oil

2. 1 Tablespoon Coconut Oil

3. ½ Cup Orange Juice

4. 2 Teaspoons Honey, Raw

5. ½ Teaspoon Rosemary, Dried

6. 1 Cup Blueberries, Frozen

7. ½ Cup Almond Butter

8. ½ Cup Ice

Directions:

1. Just throw everything into the blender, and make sure to blend on high. A high speed blender will usually work a little better. If you don't have a powerful blender, blend the rosemary, almond butter, and coconut oil together first before adding the rest of the ingredients to make sure you get a smooth texture.

Chapter 6. Almond Oil Soap For Gifts & Use

Sweet almond oil soap is great for your skin. You already know that sweet almond oil can help you with beauty, but it can help you in your hygiene routine as well. Of course, there are many different types of soaps that you can make, and you can even decorate them as gifts. It's all from the recipe to the packaging, and everything in between. Many people will even let flowers and herbs top it to give it that nice look, but it's not necessary. Your almond oil can be simple and plain, and it can still be helpful to your skin, stress levels, and mood.

Soap #1 The Basic Bar

This is just the most basic almond oil soap that you can make. It's relatively easy to make, and it doesn't take that many ingredients. It won't exactly look pretty, but it'll do the job of nourishing your skin and making sure that you look younger, healthier, and smell even better.

Ingredients:

1. 90 Grams Sweet Almond Oil

2. 326 Grams Distilled Water

3. 126 Grams Lye

4. 270 Grams Palm Oil

5. 270 Grams Olive Oil

6. 270 Grams Coconut Oil

Directions:

1. Make your lye solution by measuring out the water you need and the lye you need. The lye should be in a separate container. Remember that you can never add the water to the lye. Always add the lye to the water when making your solution. Make sure it's mixed and set it aside.

2. Pour your hot lye solution onto the hard oils, and stir it while it melts.

3. Next, you're going to want to add in your soft oils. Mix and pour it into a soap mold.

This is the room temperature method of making soap, and it still needs to wait four to six weeks before the soap is ready to use.

Soap #2 Chocolate Almond Soap

If you're looking for a soap that is a great gift, then this is the soap for you. It's great for spring time, and remember that you need to let them sit for three to four weeks before making them. The bars are going to darken when they cure, and it'll often be extremely fragrant. This delicious smelling bar moisturizes your skin and gives you a relaxing scent you can be happy with.

Ingredients:

1. 225 Grams Olive Oil

2. 180 Grams Almond Oil

3. 270 Grams Coconut Oil

4. 90 Grams mango Seed Butter

5. 90 Grams Cocoa Butter

6. 45 Grams Castor Oil

7. 32 Grams Goat's Milk, Frozen

8. 127 Grams Lye

9. 2 Teaspoons Cocoa

10. 4 Tablespoons Almond Oil

11. 2 Tablespoons Mokalata Fragrance Oil

Directions:

1. Start by making your lye solution, and remember to wear safety goggles as well as rubber gloves. To do this pour the amount of lye you need into a mason jar, making sure to not get any stray pieces anywhere. Slowly add the lye to the amount of water that your recipe calls for. Make sure that it doesn't splash. Never add the water to the lye, or it can explode

in the pitcher in a dangerous and volcano-like fashion. So always add the lye to the water.

2. The cold process method which this soap is made with is great if it's your first time, and you need to start by melting your oils together, blending the soft and hard oils together.

3. Next, blend in your lye solution carefully. They need to be brought to similar temperatures to do this, so bring them to about 90 degrees.

4. Once combined, you can whisk or use a stick blender until its thick, and then you pour it into your soap mold.

5. You have to wait about four to six weeks before you can use this soap.

Soap #3 A Rosemary Dill Bar

Rosemary and dill is a clean scent that can be used in the kitchen. It's actually great if you want to keep your hands soft and smooth, but it will also rid you of any smells that linger on your hands, such as from garlic or onions. Remember that you are using the cold processing method with this soap.

Ingredients:

1. 4 Ounces Sweet Almond Oil

2. 6 Ounces Coconut Oil

3. 10 Ounces Palm Oil

4. 12 Ounces Olive Oil

5. 12 Ounces Distilled Water

6. 4Ounces Lye

7. 1 Tablespoon Rosemary, Ground

8. ½ Tablespoon Dill, Ground

9. ½ Tablespoon Coffee Grounds

10. 1 Tablespoon Rosemary Essential Oil

Directions:

1. Remember to take special care when using lye because it is dangerous, and as stated in previous soap recipes make your lye solution. Make sure that you are adding the lye to the water. Let it cool to a hundred degrees.

2. Reserve a half an ounce of sweet almond oil, and then heat all of the oil together.

3. Add the essential oils to the reserved almond oil.

4. When the oils have cooled to about a hundred degrees, slowly add in the lye solution to it, stirring constantly so that it combines well.

5. Wait for it to thicken, which is often referred to as tracing, and then runa line of mix over the top of the solution. Add the sweet almond oil that has been mixed

with the essential oil, and then add the coffee grounds, dill and rosemary.

6. Pour it all into the molds that you have put aside, and it should set in twenty-four hours, but you shouldn't use it for three weeks. It should cure.

Remember:

Remember to keep lye out of the reach of children. It is a dangerous chemical, and if you get it on you, then you will experience a chemical burn. You should measure everything carefully when making soap. After these soaps are cured, they are safe to use, and they're easy to make in the meantime. They make great gifts, and will usually make at least six bars. However, it does depend on the type of soap molds that you are using.

You can cut them to any size if you are using just a block mold. However, there are soap molds that will give you any shape that you want, making them even more fun to use. Remember that you can actually ad flowers or herbs to the top of them before they cure to give them that extra look that promises beauty along with the benefits that almond oil has to offer. Mint, rosemary, rose petals, and lavender are very popular to add to the top of soaps, especially almond oil soaps.

Chapter 7. Almond Oil for Various Ailments

Almond oil can help with various ailments, and you'll find it can help with everything from sore muscles to dandruff. It all depends on the way you're using it, so make sure to follow these directions, and it'll be easy to make sure that you're getting everything you can out of the almond oil you've bought. If you use it too often, then you should buy in bulk to make sure that you can use it to help with various ailments and almond oil hacks.

Solution #1 A Headache Solution

Almond oil can be great to help sooth your headache away, and it's incredibly easy to use. You can actually use almond oil on your own, but it works a little better if you have the essential oils listed below. This is a simple solution, and your headache will be gone after one application or at least severely lessened.

Ingredients:

1. 2-4 Drops Peppermint Essential Oil

2. 5-6 Drops Lavender Essential Oil

3. 1 Teaspoon Sweet Almond Oil

Directions:

1. Mix all ingredients together, and then rub on your temples for about ten to fifteen minutes to get immediate relief.

Solution #2 Sore Muscle Relief

You can get relief from your sore muscles fast with almond oil as well. Of course, you'll find that it is mostly used for a carrier oil, but it can relax you enough that you make sure not to tense your muscles when you're trying to feel better. The essential oils will also help. Lavender oil is known for pain relief, and sandalwood can help to stop muscle spasming. The rosemary essential oil is great for relieving both muscle and joint pain.

Ingredients:

1. 5 Tablespoons Sweet Almond Oil

2. 5-8 Drops Rosemary Essential Oil

3. 8-10 Drops Sandalwood Essential Oil

4. 5-6 Drops Lavender Essential Oil

Directions:

1. Mix everything together, and then make sure to massage it into your sore muscles.

Solution #3 Indigestion Help

Indigestion is something that everyone faces every once in a while, but there's no reason to deal with it. You can fight indigestion with sweet almond oil. With the peppermint oil, which helps with indigestion as well, then you'll be able to feel better quicker. This is not a recipe that you're meant to ingest.

Ingredients:

1. 3-4 Drops Peppermint Essential Oil

2. 1 Teaspoon Almond Oil

Directions:

1. Mix it together, and rub it on your abdomen. It should help with indigestion immediately. However, if you want to make something that you do take orally, then just add a half a teaspoon of

peppermint extract with a teaspoon of almond oil and take like that.

Solution #4 Chapped Lips

Almond oil can be applied directly to chapped lips, and it'll help on its own. However, the salve that you find below helps a little more. There are many different reasons that you'd want to consider chapped lips an ailment, and it can lead to cold sores if it's not taken care of. Not to mention that it's painful, so it's important that you use almond oil to take care of the problem before it gets too bad.

Ingredients:

1. 4 Tablespoons Sweet Almond Oil

2. 2 Teaspoons Beeswax, Grated

3. 2 Teaspoons Shea Butter

4. ¼ Teaspoon Vitamin E Oil

5. 10 Drops Chamomile Essential oil

6. 3 Drops Lavender Essential Oil

7. 5-7 drops Peppermint Essential Oil

Directions:

1. Melt your almond oil, shea butter, and beeswax together over low heat in a double boiler.

2. Remove it from the heat, and then add in your vitamin E oil, stirring before you finish and add in your essential oil.

3. Put it in lip balm tubes, letting it cool before you store it in a dark place after labeling. This can actually last two to three years, and you apply it like you would normal lip balm, but it'll help to heal any sores that you have on your lips as well.

Solution #5 Almond Oil Lotion for Sunburn

You can actually help to heal up your sunburn if you make an almond oil lotion, and it makes it easy to help make sure that your sunburn heals without any problem. It can even help with the pain because each ingredient has been picked to make sure that your skin is soothed from the burn and yet healing.

Ingredients:

1. ½ Cup Aloe Vera Gel

2. ½ Cup Almond Oil

3. 2 Carrots, Peeled & Grated

4. 1 Teaspoon Beeswax

5. 2 Teaspoons Emulsifying Wax

6. 1 Teaspoon Vitamin C Powder

7. ½ Teaspoon Vitamin E Oil

Directions:

1. The carrots should be grated up fine, and then you will want to place them in a pan with your almond oil. They should be heated gently in the oil for about twenty-five to thirty minutes.

2. You are then going to want to strain your carrots out, adding the liquid back to the pan, and then add your waxes. Stir it all while they melt, and then add in the vitamin C powder, vitamin E oil, and your aloe vera.

3. Make sure to whisk until its smooth and creamy, taking it off heat to do so.

4. Pour it into a jar and let it cool. It should thicken, and then you can apply it to sunburn generously. It can keep up to two months when refrigerated.

Solution #6 Another Sunburn Solution

You may not always have time to make a cream for your sunburn because no one can think ahead all of the time. Of course, almond oil can help to provide you a quick remedy as well, with a lot more common ingredients. There's no reason that you should have to deal with your sunburn.

Ingredients:

1. 1 Cup Milk, Chilled

2. 2 Teaspoons Almond Oil

3. 3 Teaspoons Peppermint Extract

4. 2 Teaspoons Honey, Raw

Directions:

1. Pop all of your ingredients into a blender, and make sure to blend until everything is mixed. Keep it cool, and then apply it to your sunburn. You can actually soak in the ingredients, but most people will just soak a wash cloth in it, laying it over their sunburn.

2. You should notice relief immediately, but it will also help you to heal your sunburn quickly. If you want added benefits, add a

teaspoon of vitamin E oil if you have it on hand. Do this two or three times daily until your sunburn is gone.

Solution #7 High Blood Pressure

You can just add almond oil into your diet if you want to make sure that you're using almond oil to help control your high blood pressure, but you'll find that this remedy works a little better. You'll want to take it once every morning, and it'll help you to control your high blood pressure over time. You can put it in water as well, but with milk this is a high blood pressure drink that is sure to help. Cinnamon will help you to lower your high blood pressure as well, and it's great to pair the two.

Ingredients:

1. 1 Teaspoon Sweet Almond Oil

2. ½ Teaspoon Cinnamon

3. 1 Teaspoon Honey, Raw

4. 4 Ounces Milk, Cold

Directions:

1. Mix everything together, and then drink every morning.

Chapter 8. Bonus Tips & Uses for Almond Oil

Remember that almond oil is a great way to make sure that you stay healthy, and it can help you with a variety of things. Adding it into your diet is going to be a big help, so make sure to keep sweet almond oil on hand. There is no reason that you should need bitter almond oil, so keep the toxic version out of your home. Instead, remember that sweet almond oil is a healthy substitution for many cooking oils.

Look for Food Grade:

It's important that you look for a food grade almond oil. This is not bitter almond oil. It's important that when you buy almond oil to use, you can use it for every remedy that has been found in this book from your hair to your health. Edible almond oil can do it all, and if you're unsure, don't buy it. Always ask the manufacturer if necessary to make sure you're getting the right grade of almond oil.

Store It Well:

You also need to store your almond oil well if you want to be able to continue to use it and reap the benefits. You need it to be kept in a cool and dark place so that the nutritional benefits are still present. Otherwise, your oil can actually taste rancid or bad, and should not be eaten. Even if you store your almond oil correctly, you will need to watch out for the expiration date. You should not use almond oil past its expiration date because this can also pose a risk to your health.

Just Apply It:

Even if you aren't going to make a lotion or salve anytime soon, you can just apply almond oil to your hair and skin to get some of the benefits. Be careful when applying it too regularly on its own to your face, though. Almond oil is an oil, and can clog pores if you are putting too much on. This is why a little goes a long ways, but it's important that you use almond oil if you want to get better, younger looking skin. It'll help to provide a glow and moisturize your skin no matter where you put it.

Throw It In:

Even if you aren't going to make complicated almond oil recipes, you should still use it because almond oil has a lot to offer. Sweet almond oil can be thrown into almost every recipe if you put in just a teaspoon or so. Replace your cooking oil, and even put it into any smoothie you make. It shouldn't change the taste, but it's going to help make sure that you're using it regularly so that you can reap the benefits that it offers. You can even just take a teaspoon a day.

Share the Help:

You can even share the help that almond oil has to offer if you make sure that you make up the recipes shown above, such as the salves and creams, and you'll be able to give them as gifts. Many people love a helpful salve or lotion to help them get through the day. If you know they have sore muscles, make sure to make a salve that helps with sore muscles using almond oil, and just package it in a pretty jar with a ribbon and card to make the perfect gift. Almond oil offers a lot of solutions, and you should always pass the love along to make sure that you're not the only one you know reaping the benefits that almond oil offers you.

It's a Base Oil:

Remember that almond oil is a base oil, and you'll want to use it when a recipe requires a base oil. It can commonly be referred to as a carrier oil as well, and that will help to make sure that you're getting almond oil added into your daily routine. For example, if you are using essential oils for one reason or another, you can pair them with a carrier oil, and you shouldn't have to reach for the olive oil. Almond oil will help to act as your carrier oil and add its own benefits.

Things to Remember:

Its light colored and can be added to vegetable dips, salad and just to cook in. it can help with your cardiovascular health as well, and that's because it'll offer you protection against various cardiovascular disease, and it can reduce your cholesterol levels when you're using it in your diet regularly. It's also a good way to get your vitamin E which will help you protect your body from free radicals which are linked to chronic illness as well as aging.

Almond oil is low in saturated fats and it is high in monounsaturated fats, which are healthy for you. Saturated fats have negative effects on your healthy, and they can even increase your risk of cancer, heart disease, and even negatively affect your bone healthy. However, monounsaturated fats are going to have the opposite effect on your body, helping you to stay healthy and fit. They can even help to keep your blood sugar levels

regular, which will help you to reduce your risk
of having type 2 diabetes.